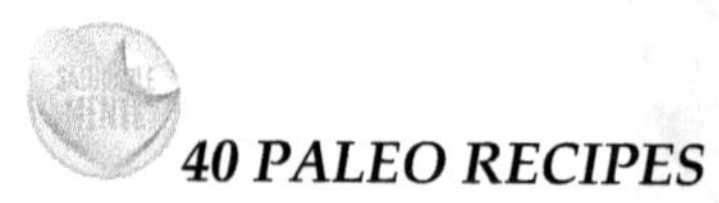 **40 PALEO RECIPES**

40 PALEO RECIPES

Index

Lean meat stew in slow cooker

Mini Mushroom Quiche

The best marinade for beef

Tasty lamb meatballs

Italian sausage pizza

Ham and egg cups

Mini Beef and Bacon Bread

The best fried meat

Broccoli and Beef Soup

Spiced vegetable and meat soup

Berry and coconut waffle

Roast chicken with lemon pepper

Bison meat burgers

Pesto fillets

Desserts

Sweet potato ice cream

Apple and beet juice

Cranny's Quotes and Walnut Bars

Cranny Banana Brownies

Coconut Pikelets

Sweet Pumpkin Waffles

Breakfast cereals

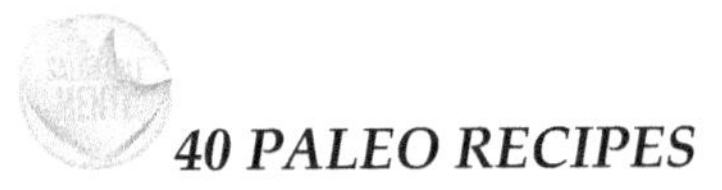

Introduction

The Paleo diet is based on the foods that the Hunter/Gatherer ate in the Paleolithic era. They are basic, simple and healthy foods. If you can't eat it, growing it or harvesting it is not part of the Paleo diet.

It includes organic farm-raised meats, fish, shellfish, seeds, nuts, vegetables, fruits and oils.

Natural and whole organic foods are full of nutrients in the right combination for our body's needs.

There is little disease when the body has all the right proteins, carbohydrates, fats,

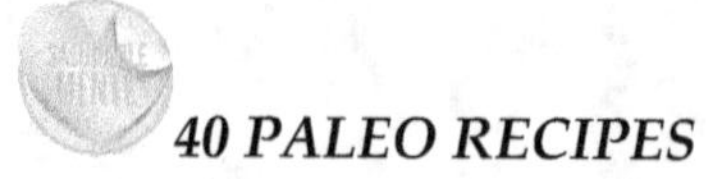

vitamins and minerals. This is the diet for the seriously healthy and all who love good food. These recipes are full of flavor, easy to make, and very good for you. Each one can be easily adapted to your pantry and preferences.

Enjoy!

Vegetables

Japanese Ratatouille

Serves: 4

Ingredients

1 tablespoon fresh oregano, chopped

1 tablespoon of fresh basil, chopped

¼ teaspoon cayenne pepper

Pepper and salt to taste

¼ cup of cooking oil

2 Japanese aubergines

6 tomatoes

2 peppers.

4 cloves of garlic, chopped

1 onion, chopped

2 courgettes

Instructions

1. Vegetable cubes

2. Heat the oil in a soup pot

3. Sauté garlic, onion 1 minute

4. Add the vegetables 1 minute

5. Add the rest of the ingredients and simmer until the eggplant is soft. Serve with your favorite meat

Cooking tips

To prepare the aubergine, peel and cut it finely, place it in a sieve and sprinkle it with salt, all the bitter juices will come out. After about twenty minutes, rinse well and then cook.

Variation

Use rosemary instead of oregano and basil

Use sun-dried tomatoes

Add sausage or chopped salami

Lemon vinaigrette

Serves: ½ cup

Ingredients

Pepper and salt to taste

2 teaspoons lemon juice

1 teaspoon lemon peel

2 tablespoons of vinegar

½ cup of virgin olive oil

Instructions

1. Place all ingredients in a glass jar with a tight-fitting lid

2. Shake well to combine

3. Use as a salad dressing

Cooking tips

Use fresh or store up to 1 week in the refrigerator, shake well before use.

Variation

Add a clove of minced garlic or some cumin

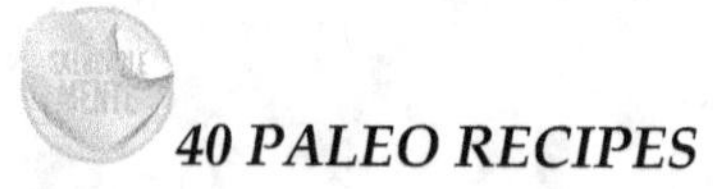

Pumpkin chips

Serves: 2

Ingredients

Pepper and salt to taste

2 teaspoons of freshly chopped herbs

¼ cup of cooking oil

4 cups thinly sliced buttercup or similar pumpkin

Instructions

1. Preheat the oven to 425F

2. Mix all ingredients in a bowl

3. Spread the pumpkin pieces on a tray in a single layer

4. Bake for 20-30 minutes, until crisp

5. Serve hot with your favorite sauce

Cooking tips

Mix the oil and seasonings/ herbs before mixing them with pumpkin pieces to evenly distribute the flavors.

Variation

Use potatoes

Add smoked paprika or pieces of bacon for more flavor.

Eggplant stuffed with sea

Serves: 4

Ingredients

3 tablespoons of oil

1 beaten egg

1 tablespoon of fish sauce

2 tablespoons of red curry paste

¼ cup chopped coriander

½ cup chopped scallions

4 cloves of garlic, minced

1 tablespoon of grated ginger

1 chopped pepper

12 ounces of raw peeled shrimp

1 large aubergine

Instructions

1. Preheat the oven to 400F

2. Cut the aubergine in half lengthwise, mark the cutting surface

3. Brush all sides with oil

4. Bake the skin for about 15 minutes

5. Turn and cook until tender

6. Remove and allow to cool

7. Remove the meat and dice

8. Fry in oil at medium heat

9. Add the pepper, garlic and ginger

10. Stir in coriander and onions, cook slightly

11. Transfer to a bowl

12. Stir the curry, sauce, egg and shrimp

13. Mixing spoon in aubergine cans

14. Bake at 350F until the filling is ready

15. Garnish with coriander

Cooking tips

Be careful when removing the cooked eggplant, not to puncture the skin.

Variation

Replace shrimp with chopped seafood or sausage/salami. Use browned pork and add some fresh chopped rosemary.

Grilled mushrooms with garlic

Serves: 2

Ingredients

2 tablespoons of oil

1 tablespoon balsamic vinegar

1 teaspoon of salt

1 teaspoon freshly ground pepper

1 teaspoon of paprika

½ teaspoon crushed coriander seeds

½ teaspoon onion powder

½ teaspoon garlic powder

3 cloves of garlic, minced

12 button mushrooms

Instructions

1. Heat the oil in a frying pan

2. Stir the spices and garlic

3. When it is slightly brown, add the vinegar and simmer for 1 minute

Cooking advice

Don't wash the mushrooms, clean them with a damp cloth. Keep the mushrooms in a brown paper bag

Variation

Add the finely chopped onion and bacon

Add the diced scallops

Garlic, mint and zucchini

Serves: 2

Ingredients

Pepper and salt to taste

2 tablespoons chopped fresh mint

The peel and juice of half a lemon

2 cloves of garlic, minced

1 tablespoon of cooking oil

2 large zucchini, sliced

Instructions

1. Heat the oil in a frying pan

2. Light brown zucchini

3. Add the ingredients, except mint, and cook for two minutes

4. Add the mint and cook for two minutes.

5. Serve hot with your favorite meat dish

Cooking tips

Use a large marrow

Variation

Cover the zucchini with spices and oil and grill, turning to cook through using rosemary, sage, thyme or oregano instead of mint.

Oven-roasted cauliflower recipe

Serves: 2-4

Ingredients

Pepper and salt to taste

½ top oil

1 tablespoon of curry powder

1 cauliflower head, cut into florets

Instructions

1. Simmer the cauliflower in water until tender

2. Drain and mix the oil and curry powder

3. Transfer to a baking tray lined with aluminum foil

4. Grill for ten minutes, or until golden brown

Cooking tips

Add the cauliflower to the boiling water, then simmer

Variation

Use broccoli instead of cauliflower

Use cumin and coriander instead of curry powder

Breakfast Hash

Serves: 2

Ingredients

Pepper and salt to taste

¼ teaspoon cayenne pepper

1 clove of garlic, minced

½ chopped onion

½ sweet potato, grated

2 eggs

Butter

Instructions

1. Melt the butter in the pan

2. Lightly sauté garlic, onion and potato

3. Adding spices to taste

4. Stir the eggs and cover

5. Cook 2-3 minutes

Cooking tips

Heat the pan halfway, not too hot or the eggs will burn

Variation

Using the potato instead of the sweet potato

Add the shredded leftover meat

Use the leftovers from the previous night, fry lightly, add the egg and cook

Sweet Cinnamon Fries

Serves: 4

Ingredients

Cinnamon

Vegetable oil

4 cups of thinly sliced sweet potatoes

Instructions

1. Heat the oil to medium/high temperature until the bubbles rise to the surface (about 250F)

2. Cook one cup of chips at a time

3. Turn frequently, cook until crisp and golden brown

4. Remove to drain on a paper towel-lined plate

5. Serve with cinnamon sprinkled on top

Cooking tips

To see if the oil is hot enough, try putting a chip, if it rises to the surface with a lot of little bubbles around it, it's ready.

Variation

Use potatoes, carrots or pumpkin chips

Sprinkle smoked paprika and sea salt over the chips. Serve with avocado sauce.

Baking

Almond and buckwheat rolls

Serves: 12

Ingredients

½ cup of sliced almonds

½ teaspoon vanilla essence

1/3 cup vegetable oil

¼ cup of honey

1 egg

1 cup almond milk

½ tablespoon of cocoa powder

½ teaspoon baking soda

1 teaspoon baking powder

¼ teaspoon salt

1 heaped cup of light buckwheat flour

Instructions

1. Preheat the oven to 375F

2. Line a 12-cup muffin tray

3. Beat vanilla, oil, honey, egg and milk

4. Sift the cocoa, baking powder, salt and flour

5. Mix well

6. Stir the almonds

7. The dough from the spoon in the bread tray

8. Bake for about twenty minutes or until firm in the center

9. Let it sit for ten minutes and then cool it on a tray

Cooking tips

Don't mix it up too much, because the cupcakes will come out hard

Variation

Omit the cocoa and replace it with instant coffee

Replace cut almonds with chocolate chips or dried cranberries

Carrot and banana rolls

Serves: 12

Ingredients

¾ cup of chopped nuts

1 ½ cups grated carrot

¼ cup melted coconut oil

1 teaspoon of vinegar

3 eggs

3 ripe bananas

1 cup of chopped dates

1 tablespoon cinnamon

1 teaspoon of salt

2 teaspoons baking soda

2 cups almond flour

Instructions

1. Preheat the oven to 350F

2. Line a muffin tray with paper cups

3. Mix oil, vinegar, eggs, bananas and dates in a food processor

4. Click on the dry ingredients until they are mixed

5. Fold the carrots and nuts.

6. Place the spoon on the prepared tray

7. Bake about 25 minutes

8. Cooling in a tray

Cooking tips

Bake in the middle of the oven to prevent the bottom from burning

Use macadamia nuts, walnuts or pecans

Variation

Use zucchini instead of carrots

Blueberries or chopped apricots instead of dates

Cranny Buns

Serves: 16

Ingredients

1 tablespoon of orange peel

1 teaspoon of salt

1 egg

1 teaspoon baking soda

2 tablespoons of honey

3 tablespoons of grated coconut

½ cup of blueberries

2 cups almond flour

Instructions

1. Preheat the oven to 375F

2. Mix the honey and the egg

3. Add the remaining ingredients

4. Briefly knead and shape the buns

5. Bake on a floured or greased baking sheet for about ten minutes or until well cooked

6. Fresh on a shelf

Cooking tips

Make buns about ½ thick

Variation

Use chopped dates, dried apricots or sultanas

Replace coconut with coconut flour, add 1/3 cup fresh chopped herbs and omit the shell

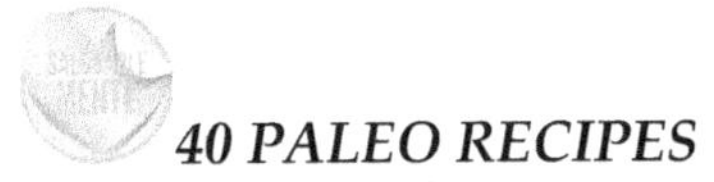

Walnut and banana bread

Serves: 12

Ingredients

¼ top oil

1 tablespoon of honey

1 tablespoon of vanilla essence

3 eggs

3 medium bananas

1 teaspoon baking soda

¼ teaspoon salt

1 ½ cups of ground nuts

¼ cup coconut flour

Instructions

1. Preheat the oven to 350F

2. Grease an 8x4 inch bread pan

3. In a food processor, mix oil, honey, vanilla, eggs and bananas

4. Mix with baking soda, salt and walnut flour

5. Pour into the prepared pan

6. Bake for about 1 hour

7. Allow to cool before turning and cutting

Cooking tips

Use frozen and thawed bananas, very moist, fresh bread

Variation

Use 2 cups almond flour instead of coconut and nuts Add ½ cup chopped nuts

Buckwheat Sandwich Wraps

Serves: 8

Ingredients

1 cup of hot water

2 tablespoons of vegetable oil

2 eggs

½ teaspoon salt

½ teaspoon baking powder

1 cup light buckwheat flour

Instructions

1. Beat all ingredients into a fine dough

2. Warming up a pan in the med-high

3. Cook in half-cup quantities, turning the pan to cover the entire surface

4. Turn after two minutes

5. Cook both sides until golden brown

Cooking tips

Making sandwich wrappers

Cut into triangles and eat with sauce

Cover with your favorite vegetable salad and fresh meat

Variation

Add ½ cup fresh chopped herbs for batter; chives, rosemary, thyme, oregano

Add some chopped garlic and chives or onion powder Add a tablespoon of roasted cumin seeds

Meats

Grilled chicken with herbs

Serves: 4

Ingredients

1/3 cup vegetable oil

3 tablespoons of vinegar

¼ teaspoon salt

1 tablespoon freshly ground pepper

1 bay leaf

2 cloves of garlic, minced

¼ cup chopped scallions

4 tablespoons of chopped parsley

¼ cup chopped oregano

4 tablespoons of chopped rosemary

2 ½ pounds of chicken breast

Instructions

1. Mix herbs, pepper and salt in a bag

2. Add the chicken and shake well to cover

3. Sit the marinated chicken in the refrigerator for at least one hour

4. Turn the oven to the grill and cook the chicken

5. Serve with sauce and your favorite vegetables

Cooking tips

Prepare the chicken marinade the day before and store it in the refrigerator. Roast the chicken at 450°F for about 20 minutes and then grill it to brown

Variation

Use grass-fed beef instead of chicken. Add a little of your favorite sauce and a teaspoon of brown sugar for marinade

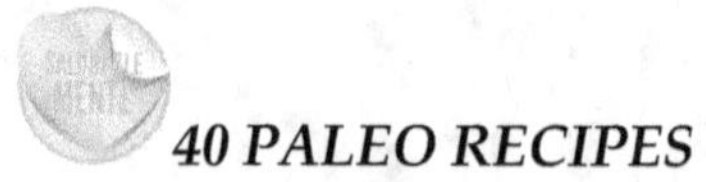

Marinade Drum Sticks

Serves: 4

Ingredients

6 sticks

1 teaspoon of salt

2 cloves of garlic, minced

1 tablespoon of vinegar

1/2 cup of water

1/2 cup chipotle peppers in adobo sauce

Instructions

1. Mix the peppers in the sauce with water, in a blender

2. Rub the chicken and refrigerate for 1-12 hours

3. Heat the oven to 400F

4. Bake in a covered dish for about 45 minutes, or until cooked

5. Ending up under the grill

Cooking tips

Cook the thighs until they are well cooked

Use 1 can of peppers and the same amount of water, use ½ cup and freeze the rest in ½ cup portions for later use

Variation

Using steaks instead of chicken

Replace peppers with your favorite sauce

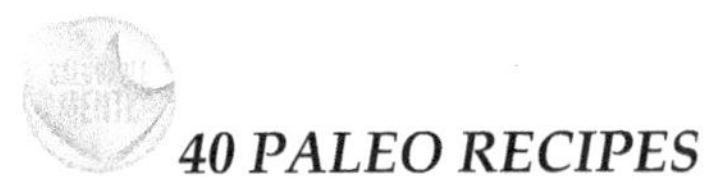

Curried Chicken and Vegetable Soup

Serves: 6

Ingredients

1 ½ pints of chicken broth

1 tablespoon of grated ginger

3 tablespoons of sauce

2-3 cups of finely chopped vegetables 1 cup of shredded curried chicken

2 cloves of garlic, minced

½ onion, chopped

1 tablespoon of vegetable oil

Instructions

1. Sauté ginger, garlic and onion in oil in a large skillet

2. Add the vegetables and chicken, two minutes

3. Stir the broth, sauce and simmer until the vegetables are tender

4. Serve hot

Cooking tips

Using leftover chicken

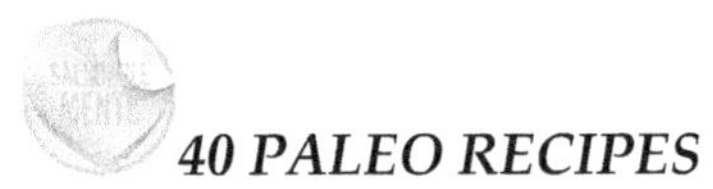

Variation

Use regular chicken and add 1 tablespoon curry paste and ½ teaspoon honey

Use turkey or duck and use red wine vinegar

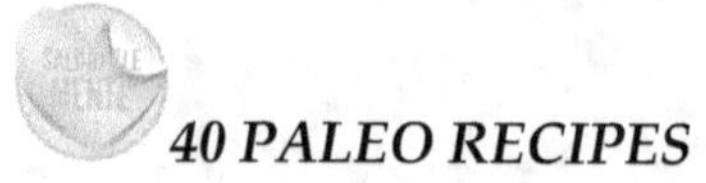

Turkey sausage casserole

Serves: 12

Ingredients

1 ½ onion, chopped

2 chopped peppers

12 eggs

1 pound of turkey sausage, chopped

Pepper and salt to taste

½ cup of chopped mushrooms

1 tablespoon of oil

2 tablespoons of chopped parsley

2 tablespoons of chopped chives, leeks or green onions

Instructions

1. Preheat the oven to 350F

2. Heat the oil in a frying pan

3. Brown sausage

4. Season to taste and pour into the baking dish

5. Sauté onions, mushrooms and peppers

6. Spread over the sausage on the baking tray

7. Beat the eggs with herbs in a bowl

8. Pour over the sausages and vegetables

9. Cook until ready, about 45 minutes

Cooking tips

Great for freezing, make an extra!

Variation

Using pork sausages

Use the shredded chicken

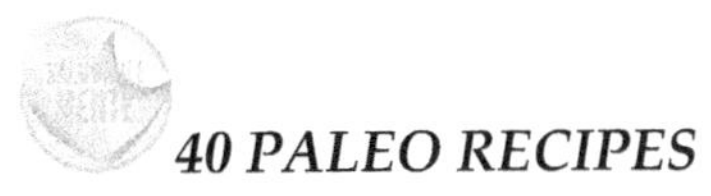

Habanero Chicken

Serves: 6

Ingredients

2 ½ pounds of chicken breast

Pepper and salt

1/3 cup of vinegar

1 cup diced tomatoes

2 tablespoons orange juice

1 teaspoon orange peel

2 cloves of minced garlic

1 onion, chopped

2 tablespoons of annatto paste

1 tablespoon of habanero sauce

Instructions

1. Mix all the ingredients together

2. Leave in the refrigerator for at least 1 hour

3. Fry in vegetable oil until cooked and serve hot.

Cooking tips

Make the marinade the night before and leave it in the fridge

Variation

Cook a whole chicken in broth and use the meat instead of the raw chicken breast. Use the cooking water to make the soup

Skip the habanero sauce for the children's meal

Lean meat stew in slow cooker

Serves: 6

Ingredients

Pepper and salt to taste

½ teaspoon of paprika

½ teaspoon cumin

1 teaspoon fresh thyme, chopped

1 teaspoon fresh rosemary, chopped

1 teaspoon freshly chopped sage

1 ½ pints of meat broth

1 pint of diced tomatoes

2 chopped peppers

2 cloves of garlic, minced

2 chopped onions

1 pound of minced lean meat

Instructions

1. Heat the oil in a soup pot

2. Browning the meat, removing the meat

3. Sauté onions and garlic

4. Add the peppers and stir-fry briefly

5. Add the browned beef and the remaining ingredients

6. Transfer to electric pot and cook 2-2 ½ hours, until meat is tender

Cooking tips

Stir the spices and herbs in the oil before cooking the meat to spread the flavor evenly. Cook on a covered plate in the oven at 350F until tender, instead of an electric cooker

Variation

Using chicken and chicken broth

Add 2 or 3 cups of finely chopped vegetables

Mini Mushroom Quiche

Serves: 12

Ingredients

Pepper to taste

12 cherry tomatoes

4 pieces of fried bacon

2 ounces of mushrooms

8 eggs

¼ cup freshly chopped herbs

Instructions

1. Preheat the oven to 350F

2. Grease a 12-cup muffin tray

3. Beat the eggs

4. Chop the mushrooms, the bacon, the tomatoes, the season

5. Put a small egg in each cup of bread

6. Sprinkle the filling

7. Put a little more egg on top

Cooking tips

Cooking the meat before putting it in mini quiches

Variation

Add grated carrot, zucchini or grated spinach to quiches

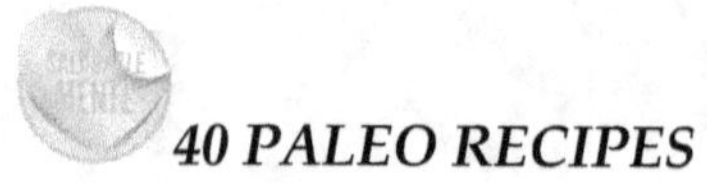

The best marinade for beef

Serves: 4

Ingredients

1 pound of cooked and minced meat

¼ teaspoon mustard powder

¼ teaspoon pepper

1 teaspoon of dried thyme

1 teaspoon dried rosemary

½ teaspoon salt

1 clove of garlic, minced

½ chopped onion

1 tablespoon of Worcestershire

1 tablespoon of honey

3 tablespoons of tomato paste

1 cup of vinegar

Instructions

1. Simmer all ingredients except meat for ten minutes

2. Add the meat and let it simmer covered for about ten minutes

3. Serve hot with mashed potatoes and steamed vegetables

Cooking tips

Brown the raw meat in oil and then simmer it in the sauce until it is cooked

Variation

Use shredded chicken or pork

Use the barbecue sauce

Tasty lamb meatballs

Serves: 5

Ingredients

¼ teaspoon cinnamon

¼ teaspoon black pepper

½ teaspoon ground cumin

1 teaspoon of ground coriander

1 teaspoon of salt

1 egg

1 tablespoon fresh mint, chopped

1 tablespoon of freshly chopped coriander

2 cloves of garlic, minced

½ onion, chopped

1 pound of lamb, chopped

Instructions

1. Preheat the oven to 375F

2. Mix all the ingredients together

3. Form meatballs the size of a tablespoon

4. Bake on a plate with a little cooking oil for ten minutes

5. Turn the meatballs, cook them for 5 to 10 minutes, until they are well cooked.

Cooking Tips

Mix the minced meat last, to obtain an even distribution of flavours

Variation

Use minced meat and chopped rosemary

Use chopped chicken and sage

Adding sesame seeds

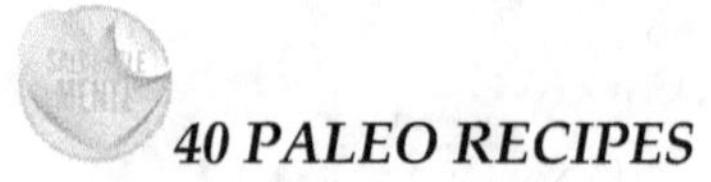

Italian sausage pizza

Serves: 8

Ingredients

Fennel seeds

oregano

½ cup cherry tomato halves

½ marinara cup

1 pepper, chopped

1 Italian sausage, sliced

4 ounces mushrooms, chopped

½ onion, chopped

1 tablespoon of olive oil

2 eggs

3 tablespoons of almond butter

1 cup almond flour

Instructions

1. Preheat the oven to 350F

2. Grease a baking tray

3. Mix in a bowl, salt, eggs, almond butter and flour

4. Knead in a dough and press it flat, on the prepared tray

5. Bake for ten minutes

6. Lightly sauté the sausage, mushrooms, onion

7. Add pepper and garlic, sauté for 1 minute

8. Spread the marinade on the crust

9. Sprinkle with sautéed vegetables and sausages

10. Sprinkle with fennel seeds and oregano

11. Bake about 25 minutes

12. When cooked, cover with cherry tomatoes

Cooking tips

The dough of the almond flour pizza is soft, be careful when transferring the slices to a plate

Variation

Use ham, bacon or chicken instead of sausages

Add olives, avocado slices or capers

Ham and egg cups

Serves: 3

Ingredients

Pepper and salt to taste

3/4 cup hollandaise sauce

1 pepper in julienne

2 cups fresh arugula

6 eggs

6 slices of ham

Instructions

1. Preheat the oven to 350F

2. Grease a 6-cup muffin tray

3. Cut each piece of ham from the center to the edge to make a cone and line the roll tray.

4. Fill each cup with an egg and season

5. Bake for about fifteen minutes

6. Briefly sauté the peppers and mix them with arugula

7. Dress the arugula and peppers with lemon vinaigrette

8. Serve the ham and egg cups on a bed of rocket salad and drizzle with hollandaise sauce

Cooking tips

Use large eggs or fill the remaining space with grated cheese or chopped parsley or onions

Variation

Line the cups with bacon

Beat the egg with the chopped onion or grated carrot and then pour it into the ham cups

Mini Beef and Bacon Bread

Serves: 4

Ingredients

Pepper to taste

2 tablespoons fresh chopped parsley

1/3 cup chopped fresh chives

2 cloves of garlic, minced

¼ cup of coconut milk

8 strips of bacon and ½ pound of chopped bacon

1 pound of minced meat

Instructions

1. Preheat the oven to 400F

2. Grease an 8-cup muffin tray

3. Mix the coconut milk, chives, garlic, pepper, chopped bacon and minced meat

4. Line muffin cups with bacon strips

5. Fill cups with minced meat mixture

6. Bake for half an hour

7. Cool and serve with parsley on top

Cooking tips

Use an electric blender to mix the minced meat ingredients

Variation

Use grated vegetables instead of ground meat

Cover with grated cheese before baking

Add an egg to the mince mixture

The best fried meat

Serves: 4

Ingredients

2 tablespoons of oil

¼ cup meat broth

Pepper and salt to taste

½ chopped onion

1 ½ teaspoons lime juice

1 teaspoon of oregano

2 cloves of garlic, minced

1 pound of minced meat

Instructions

1. Add oil to the hot pan

2. Add garlic, onion, pepper, salt and oregano

3. Add minced meat and stir to brown 1-2 minutes

4. Mix the lime juice and meat stock, pour into the pan

5. Turn down the heat and cook

6. Serve hot with your favorite vegetables

Cooking tips

Cook the meat first on a high heat for a few minutes, then on a low heat until it cooks to obtain a tender meat

Variation

Marinate the minced meat in premixed broth and spices/ herbs, in the refrigerator

Cook the minced meat in seasoned oil

Add twice the broth when it is almost cooked, mix some corn starch with some broth and stir the meat to form a sauce

Minced meat can be used for shepherd's pie, pasta or with sauce and rice

Broccoli and Beef Soup

Serves: 6

Ingredients

1 pound of chopped broccoli

1 pound of cooked meat in cubes

1 clove of garlic, minced

½ chopped onion

4 tablespoons of soy sauce

4 tablespoons freshly grated ginger

3 pints of meat stock

Instructions

1. Heat the broth over a low heat

2. Stir all the ingredients

3. Simmer until broccoli is tender

4. Serve with mashed potatoes

Cooking tips

Fry the raw meat in a little oil, then cook it over a low heat until it is well cooked, add the broth and cook according to the

Variation

Use pork, chicken or turkey and 1 pound of mixed vegetables in cubes

Add some chilies, peppers and tomatoes

Spiced vegetable and meat soup

Serves: 6

Ingredients

Pepper and salt to taste

2 tablespoons of oil

1 cup of coconut milk

2 pints of meat stock

1 tablespoon cinnamon

½ teaspoon ground cloves

½ teaspoon ground turmeric

¼ teaspoon ground nutmeg

1 tablespoon of mild curry powder

¼ cup fresh chopped parsley

1 chopped parsnip

1 chopped leek

2 chopped apples

2 chopped carrots

1 chopped potato

1 onion, chopped

1 cup chopped mixed vegetables; cauliflower, broccoli, beans, peas 2 celery sticks, chopped

1 ½ pounds of minced meat

Instructions

1. Heat the oil in a soup pot

2. Minced meat, garlic, onion

3. Add the rest of the vegetables and sauté for 1-2 minutes

4. Stir the spices and parsley

5. Add the coconut milk and meat broth

6. Simmer until vegetables are tender

7. Seasoning to taste

8. Serve hot

Cooking tips

Stir the spices in the oil before browning the meat, to obtain a uniform flavor throughout the dish Chop all the small vegetables to improve the flavor and shorten the cooking time

Variation

Use chicken, turkey, pork or lamb instead of beef. Use any fresh vegetables you have on hand

Add fresh herbs

Cover with Greek-style yogurt

Berry and coconut waffle

Serves: 4

Ingredients

¼ cup raspberries (extra for topping)

¼ cup coconut cream

1 tablespoon of honey

1 teaspoon of vanilla essence

½ teaspoon cinnamon

2 eggs

½ teaspoon baking soda

¼ cup dried coconut

1 ½ cups almond flour

Instructions

1. Heat the waffle iron

2. Mix the ingredients in a bowl

3. Cooking on the waffle iron

4. Serve with extra berries and honey for sweetening

Cooking tips

If the waffles stick together, grease the waffle iron with butter between each one. Defrost the berries in a strainer over a bowl, discard the liquid

Variation

Use blueberries or strawberries

Skip the coconut and use chopped nuts, walnuts or pecans and a little spice mix

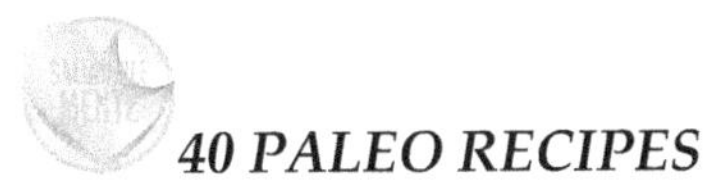

Roast chicken with lemon pepper

Serves: 4

Ingredients

Salt to taste

Lemon pepper

1 garlic clove

1 teaspoon fresh rosemary or sage

4 chicken breasts

Instructions

1. Preheat the oven for baking

2. Line a baking tray with aluminum foil

3. Sprinkle the chicken with lemon pepper and salt

4. Place the chicken on a prepared tray

5. Sprinkle with herbs and place the garlic clove in the tray

6. Grill 10-15 minutes

7. Turn and roast the other side 10-15 minutes

8. Serve when golden brown

Cooking tips

Cook at 350F on a covered plate for about 30 minutes, then brown under the grill

Variation

Use lamb chops

Cover the meat with sliced onions and your favorite sauce

Bison meat burgers

Serves: 4

Ingredients

Pepper and salt to taste

2 cloves of garlic, minced

1 egg

1 jalapeño pepper

1 tablespoon fresh rosemary, chopped

1 teaspoon fresh thyme, chopped

1 onion, chopped

1 pound bison chopped

Instructions

1. Mix all the ingredients

2. Making hamburgers

3. Fry in a medium/hot skillet until well cooked.

4. Cook both sides

5. Serve hot on hamburger buns with your favorite salad and sauce.

Cooking tips

Grill on a baking sheet with aluminum foil in the center of the oven

Variation

Use chopped chicken, pork or turkey

Form balls and use them for spaghetti and meatballs

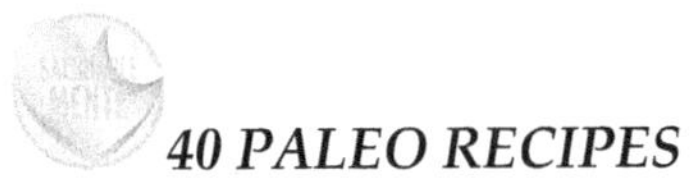

Pesto fillets

Serves: 6

Ingredients

Pepper and salt to taste

Cooking spray

2 tablespoons almond flour

2 tablespoons pesto sauce

6 tilapia fillets

Instructions

1. Preheat the oven to 400F

2. Prepare a baking tray with cooking spray

3. Arrange the fillets in the pan

4. Sprinkle remaining ingredients on top

5. Bake for ten minutes, or until well cooked

6. Serve with sweet cinnamon potatoes

Cooking tips

Put the pesto, flour and seasonings in a plastic bag, add the fish and shake it gently to cover it with flavor

Variation

First use beef steaks and marinate them in the refrigerator

Sprinkle fish with freshly grated ginger and chopped scallions before baking. Add crushed fennel seeds to season fish

Desserts

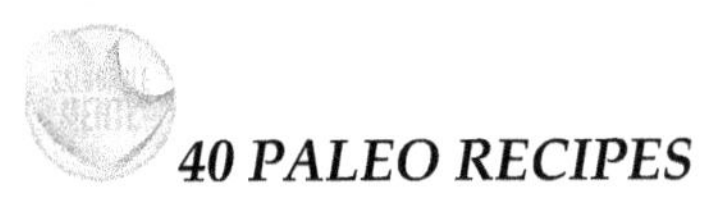 *40 PALEO RECIPES*

Sweet potato ice cream

Serves: 4

Ingredients

1/8 teaspoon salt

1/8 teaspoon nutmeg

1 teaspoon of vanilla essence

2 tablespoons cinnamon

2 egg yolks

1 tablespoon maple syrup

1 can of whole coconut milk

1 peeled and baked sweet potato

Instructions

1. Freeze the ice cream accessory overnight

2. Coconut milk and sweet potato puree in a blender

3. Mix the remaining ingredients

4. Cover the bowl with plastic wrap and freeze for two hours

5. Put the mixture in the ice cream maker and beat it for half an hour

Cooking advice

Mix the dry ingredients before mixing them with the sweet potato and milk

Variation

Replacing maple syrup with honey

Use 2 bananas instead of the sweet potato

Apple and beet juice

Serves: 1

Ingredients

2 blocks

2 beets

2 Carrots

Instructions

1. Put clean beets in a pot of water, bring to a simmer

2. After 25 minutes remove the beets and rinse in cold water

3. Peel the beets under water, trim the ends and slice

4. Peel the apples and carrots

5. Put all the ingredients in a juicer

Cooking tips

Simmer the beets in their skins to prevent all the nutrients from leaking into the water

Variation

Skip the beet and use the pineapple

Freeze the juice like a block of ice

Add celery stalks or pear slices instead of beets

Cranny's Quotes and Walnut Bars

Serves: 24 pieces

Ingredients

½ cup grated coconut

1/2 cup pitted dates

½ cup of blueberries

¼ cup of raw pistachio

¼ cup pumpkin seeds

1/2 cup walnut halves

1/2 cup of raw almonds

½ cup macadamia nuts

½ cup walnut halves

¼ cup sunflower seeds

1 teaspoon ground cinnamon

3 tablespoons of honey

1 cup of almond food

1 egg

¼ cup coconut oil

¼ cup almond butter

Instructions

1. Spread the nuts and seeds on a baking tray, roast them, stirring frequently until slightly toasted

2. Remove tray and heat oven to 350F

3. Mix the remaining ingredients, blend them well

4. Add the seeds and nuts

5. Spread on a baking tray with a spatula. Press down well

6. Bake for 10-15 minutes, until brown on the edges

7. Allow to cool

8. Cut into equal slices

9. Store at room temperature

Cooking tips

Nuts and seeds burn easily, so keep your eyes and nose on them

Bake in the center of the oven to prevent the bottom of the bars from burning

Variation

Use any mix of nuts and seeds at 2 ¾ cups Use different dried fruits; sultanas, apricots, chopped mango at 1 cup

Cranny Banana Brownies

Serves: 16

Ingredients

¼ cup of chocolate chips

¼ cup of blueberries

1 tablespoon of honey

1 tablespoon of vanilla essence

1 medium banana

16 dates

1 teaspoon cinnamon

½ cup of cocoa powder, sugar free

2 1/3 cups walnut halves

Instructions

1. Put cinnamon, cocoa and nuts in a food processor, mix gently

2. Add the banana and dates, mix

3. Add vanilla and honey, mix

4. Fold the chocolate chips and the blueberries

5. Press into a lightly greased baking dish and freeze until ready, about one hour

6. Cut into equal pieces

Cooking tips

Cover the plate or put it inside a plastic bag before freezing the

Variation

Use other dried fruits instead of dates

Use maple syrup instead of honey

Using walnuts or macadamia nuts instead of nuts

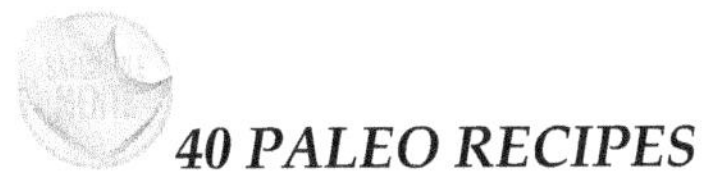

Coconut Pikelets

Serves: 4

Ingredients

2 teaspoons of vanilla essence

¼ teaspoon cinnamon

1 teaspoon baking soda

4 eggs

½ teaspoon salt

1 cup of coconut milk

1 tablespoon of honey

½ cup coconut flour

Instructions

1. Beat the milk, eggs and vanilla

2. Sift the remaining ingredients

3. Heat the oil in a frying pan

4. Place a spoonful of batter in the pan and cook until golden brown on both sides. Serve with honey or maple syrup

Cooking tips

These pikelets do not bubble, so you have to check if the cooked coconut flour is very absorbent, so you need 4 eggs

Variation

Add ½ cup of blueberries or raspberries to batter

Sweet Pumpkin Waffles

Serves: 4

Ingredients

2 teaspoons of vanilla essence

2 tablespoons pumpkin puree

1 tablespoon of oil

1 teaspoon of honey

3 eggs

½ teaspoon salt

½ teaspoon baking soda

1 teaspoon of nutmeg

½ teaspoon cloves

1 tablespoon of ground cinnamon

5 tablespoons almond flour

2 tablespoons coconut flour

Instructions

1. Beat the wet ingredients

2. Mix in the dry ingredients

3. Cooking in a well-oiled waffle iron

Cooking tips

Coconut flour is very absorbent, you just need a little

Variation

Skip the spices and pumpkin for the plain waffles

Breakfast cereals

Serves: 2

Ingredients

1 tablespoon of vanilla essence

1 tablespoon cinnamon

1 cup almond milk

2 tablespoons of oil

¼ cup of nuts

2 tablespoons of grated coconut

2 tablespoons of flax seeds

2 tablespoons pumpkin seeds

2 tablespoons of chia seeds

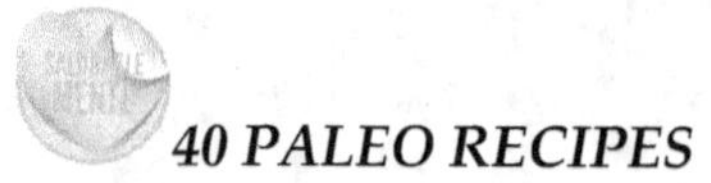

Instructions

1. Heat the oil and milk in a pan over low heat

2. Grind the remaining ingredients together

3. Stir in the milk

Cooking tips

Add more chia seeds for a thicker cereal, or less for a thinner cereal

Stir at ½ cup fresh berries, dried fruit. Add vanilla and cinnamon. Make it salty with some salt